Books by Tom

Non-Fiction

- **Pure Weight Loss: The science of detoxification and rejuvenation for life-long weight control**
  Weight loss through detoxification and rejuvenation - the future of health.

- **Nutrition-1-2-3: three diet wisdoms for losing weight, gaining energy, and reversing chronic disease**
  The basics of natural nutrition for shopping, eating and regaining your health. Throw away the fads and start enjoying health – it is as easy as 1-2-3.

Fiction

- **The President is Down** (Novel)
  The most powerful man in the world crashes in Central America where a beautiful peasant rescues him from rebels, soldiers, and himself.

- **The Last Quack** (Novel)
  Kate Turner, naturopathic physician, discovers that tripping over a dead body may be hazardous to her health, especially when the dead woman was researching the same medicinal mushroom.

- **Eco-Agent Man: the case of the vanishing moth** (Film Script)
  Nick Chronos, undercover Ecology-Agent with a bag of quirky low-tech tricks, battles a ruthless developer to save an endangered species – the Spotted Porch Light Moth.

- **Get to Know your Duck** (Play)
  The Bland family's complacent existence is scrambled when the twins bring home a two-headed duck that keeps growing... and growing...

Tom Ballard, RN, ND

After experiencing the medical-industrial complex from the inside as an emergency department nurse, Tom graduated from Bastyr University in 1982 as a doctor of naturopathic medicine. He is the founder of Pure Wellness Centers (www.PureWellnessCenters.com) in Seattle and Renton, Washington. He also founded Green Medicine, dedicated to promoting scientific, sustainable and organic medicine. Dr. Ballard has lectured internationally on nutrition, environmental detoxification, thyroid function, weight loss, and combating chronic disease. He has been published in Sound Consumer, Naturopathic News and Reviews, Health Issues Quarterly, Naturopathic Digest, and Well Being Journal. He is available for speaking and classes. Tom lives in Seattle with his pet gooey duck, Bob.

Dedication
In memory of John Bastyr, ND: a man of perpetual learning

Acknowledgements
Many thanks for the valuable assistance of
hundreds of wonderful patients,
Julie Krauss-Lucas, ND and
Candace McNaughton, ND

Pure Weight Loss

The science of detoxification & rejuvenation for lifelong weight control

Copyright 2008
(Second edition 2010)

Tom Ballard, RN, ND

ISBN 1440487669

EAN-13 9781440487668

Published by
Fresh Press Books
3315 59th Ave. SW
Seattle, WA 98116
FreshPressBooks@gmail.com

The recommendations in this book have not been evaluated by the Food and Drug Administration. It is not intended to diagnose, treat, cure, or prevent any disease. It is written solely for informational and educational purposes. Please consult your healthcare professional for your specific needs.

"One of the great health tragedies of our time is that the medical-industrial complex has been selling bad advice about nutrition for 60 years, to the point where the majority of the population have lost sight of how delicious and healthy food can be. People have come to believe that the Standard American Diet, the SAD diet, is a healthy diet and it is somehow their fault for not adhering to it. The truth is that their bodies are rebelling against nutrient-poor, toxic-laden foods."

Tom Ballard, ND

Contents

Section I

Setting the record straight

1. Introduction: Weight loss for life 2
2. Who will benefit from Pure Weight Loss 3
3. Stop blaming yourself 4
4. Is this another crash diet? 5
5. Why isn't my current diet/exercise working? 6
   - Factors affecting weight loss 6

Section II

Detoxification & Rejuvenation: Keys to a healthy weight

6. Detoxification: 21st Century Medicine 9
   A. Challenges to detoxification systems 10
   B. Consequences of toxins 11
   C. Summary of detoxification 12
7. Rejuvenation: Providing optimal nutrition 13
   - Are you deficient? 14

Section III

Getting started

8. Information gathering 18
   - History, biomarkers, free radicals 18
9. Advanced testing 20
   - Toxic metals and chemicals 20

Section IV

Your Pure Weight Loss

10. What to expect from your PWL 23
11. Components of PWL program, summary 26
12. Your PWL program 28
    A. Nutritious eating guide 28
       i. Nutrition-1-2-3: Three Wisdoms 28
       ii. Twenty diet principles for weight loss 30

   iii. Meal planning 33
     o Breakfast, lunch, dinner, snacks
   iv. Common dietary mistakes 35
   v. First Choice/Last choice food reminders.36
  B. PW Meal Shakes 37
   i. Shake ingredients 37
   ii. Mixing your shake 38
   iii. Timing your shakes 39
   iv. PWL shake recipes 40
  C. Activity..43
  D. Mind/Body Detoxification Treatments 45
   - Other detoxification strategies 46
  E. PW Supplements ....……47
   - Additional supplements 48
  F. PWL program Summary 50
 13. Monitoring your progress 51

Section V
Supporting your progress

 14. Protein content of common foods 53
 15. Tasty Detox Recipes 54
 16. Coconut oil – the healthy fat 60
 17. How allergies and sensitivities affect weight loss 64
 18. Avoid unproven detoxification treatments 69
  - colonics, food baths and pads
 19. Pure Weight Loss email and phone consultations ... 73

Section VI
Conclusion & BioMarker Record

 20. Conclusion 75
 21. BioMarker Record. 77

Section I

Setting the record straight

*"Set your current beliefs about weigh loss
aside while you read this book."*

Tom Ballard, ND

1. Weight loss for life

Your goal is to lose weight and keep it off. The **Pure Weight Loss** (PWL) program is designed to help you lose fat, not muscle. Muscle loss, as occurs in most weight loss programs, leads to lowered energy and weight gain – yo-yo dieting.

Successful fat loss is simple when you:

- **Remove** environmental toxins that slow your ability to burn calories
- **Rejuvenate** your body the nutrients it requires to produce energy and control appetite.

Note that I said nothing about starvation, calorie counting, or avoiding fats. These strategies have a 95% failure rate. **Detoxification and Rejuvenation** (optimum nutrition) are the keys to weight loss for the same reason they are successful at treating chronic disease – because they address the underlying causes.

Research shows that the average person is deficient in at least three nutrients and harbors toxic metals, plastics, pesticides, solvents, and other synthetic chemicals. This combination of nutritional deficiencies and toxic burden leads to chronic fatigue, hormone imbalances, mood and memory problems, heart disease, chronic pain, and weight gain.

2. Who will benefit from *Pure Weight Loss*?

Since virtually everyone is deficient in at least three nutrients and is toxic, a program that increases nutrient density and removes toxins could potentially benefit everyone.

The *Pure Weight Loss* program is ideal for those people like my patient Linda. She came to me saying, **"I do everything right. I exercise six days a week, hard. I'm very disciplined about my diet. It drives my husband crazy to watch how little I eat. But my weight keeps going up. How can I do so much and still be 35 pounds overweight?"** When I reviewed what Linda was doing I agreed with her. She was, for the most part, following a program that should have allowed her to lose weight.

Linda's problem wasn't lack of discipline and hard work; it was nutritional deficiencies and toxins. After finding she had extremely high levels of free radicals, I tested her for heavy metals. Again she was high. The metals were triggering the free radicals which were interfering with her ability to burn fat.

Linda found, like many others have, that as she became revitalized by detoxification and rejuvenation, her weight reflected her new vitality.

The *Pure Weight Loss* program also works well for those who feel they lack the discipline to lose weight. The program is simple and takes little time. Energy levels go up quickly – this helps you to lose weight and gain inspiration.

We've also used the program to help those who are underweight.

3. Stop blaming yourself - it's the diet

Do you describe yourself as having "no will power" because you've "failed" so many diets? Maybe you follow the menus very well for a month, then fall apart and gain back every ounce you lost, plus a pound? My advice: stop blaming yourself and blame the diet.

In over 30 years of helping people lose weight I've found that it's usually not the dieter, but the diet that's weak. Here's another way to look at it: statistics show that 95% of diets don't result in permanent weight loss. Does that mean that 95% of dieters are weak-willed? Does that sound right? Let's see, most dieters hold a job, maintain a home, support loving relationships, and even raise kids, yet they're all "weak willed"? No. This is a classic case of blaming the victim.

Who benefits when you blame yourself? The diet industry and drug manufacturers.

Who loses (or rather continues to gain weight)? You.

Not only does your weight and general health suffer, but your emotional health is pummeled when you blame yourself for failing at an impossible task. You simply cannot maintain a healthy weight on the fat-promoting programs that are the bread and butter of the diet and medical industries.

Good science, statistics, and common sense prove it is not you, but the diet's fault.

4. Is this another crash diet?

Pure Weight Loss is not for the person who wants to drop 10 pounds in a week to fit into their swimming suit. **Crash weight-loss programs cause a crash in muscle and water.** This undermines metabolism and overall health. The person who loses weight with a crash program will end up regaining that weight plus more – it's almost guaranteed.

The person who excels at Pure Weight Loss recognizes that health is wealth and their weight is a reflection of their health.

We love working with farsighted patients who are farsighted enough to know that just as they gained their weight over time, it will take time to lose it. They're also willing to apply a little discipline to their life. I'm not saying you have to become "perfect" but you must realize that actions have consequences. An analogy would be Bill Gates. He did not set out on a get-rich-quick scheme. Through years of work and dedication, he built an empire. **I want you to build an empire of health.**

5. Why isn't my current diet and exercise working?

First of all, it's important to realize that you may be trying very hard, but doing the wrong things, through no fault of your own. Most people are justifiably confused by common misinformation about nutrition and weight loss. It's like you're trying to enter a window on the second floor with a ladder, but the ladder is set on the third floor. You're working hard. You're climbing the ladder every day, but you're climbing to the wrong window.

Factors affecting your ability to lose weight:

- Health problems such as low thyroid and adrenal function, allergies, poor digestion, and low levels of B vitamins. If you suspect a problem or are not losing weight, consult with your *PW* doctor. These visits are usually covered by insurance.

- Past history of fad diets. These typically lead to yo-yo dieting and increased weight gain. It sometimes takes months to undo the damage of fad diets (And yes, by fad I include all of the most popular diet programs, some that have been around for forty years)

- Low-fat, low-calorie diets, the most common weight loss strategies, don't work. While much advertised and followed, research shows they have a 95% failure rate. They result in lowered metabolism and weight gain.

- Your current exercise program may not be enough to tip the balance toward weight loss. Sometimes just a few additional minutes a day can start your fat loss.

- Water: Being well hydrated has been shown to boost metabolism by as much as 15% and help in losing fat.

- While trying hard and believing they're eating a good diet, in my experience most people are eating diets that are low in nutrients and contributing to their weight gain.

- Not enough protein. Standard nutrition textbook recommendations for protein are ¼ to ½ gram per pound of body weight. So, a 150 pound person requires between 38 and 75 grams of protein per day. This is highly variable from person to person, but a good place to start. Most people eat a much greater percentage of carbohydrates than they need. Remember, cattle are fattened with carbs, not protein.

Section II

Detoxification & Rejuvenation: Keys to a healthy weight

"The two issues that have most undermined our health are an increasingly toxic world, including the food chain, and declining levels of nutrients in our foods."

Tom Ballard, ND

6. Detoxification: 21st Century Medicine

Am I toxic?

One hundred percent of humans tested in the US, Europe and even "remote" places such as Mongolia and Antarctica show elevated levels of industrial chemicals. Contamination is so prevalent that breast milk is now considered the most chemically contaminated of all human foods. It carries concentrations of organochlorine pollutants that are 10 to 20 times higher than cows' milk. Because detoxification systems have not evolved to handle new "man made" chemicals, they are stored in tissues.

A more appropriate question is: **How toxic am I?** (See section III on testing for environmental toxins)

Is there any science behind detoxification?

Detoxification is an ongoing process in every cell of your body. It simply refers to the removal of unwanted waste. You could not live if your body stopped eliminating toxins. For instance, your lungs take in oxygen and eliminate carbon dioxide. Your kidneys send waste from your blood to your bladder. What if your kidneys stopped working? You'd be put on a dialysis machine. When the liver, the main organ of detoxification, fails, the only hope is a successful liver transplant.

Detoxification and "cleansing" (sweat lodges, laxatives, saunas, diuretics, etc) were time-honored healing methods in every culture in the world until industrial medicine became dominant.

Treatment

During the **PWL** program you will be enjoying a mild generalized detoxification. Our goal is to increase your capacity to rid your body of toxins. Detoxification, we believe, should be an ongoing process that keeps you ahead of the incoming toxins. Most people can carry on normal activities and do not experience any unwanted side effects. If you feel you need a more intensive or more specific detoxification, speak with your health practitioner about testing and advanced treatment.

Challenges to our detoxification systems:

1. **Heavy Metals**:
   Industrialization has brought us into increased contact with these toxins by inhalation, ingestion through food and water, mercury tooth fillings, treated wood, paint, and pesticides. The results have been increasing body burdens of:

   Lead   Cadmium   Arsenic   Mercury   Aluminum

2. **Low intake of nutrients used for detoxification**
   Deficiencies are due to food processing, depletion of soil and poor food choices. Detoxification cannot take place without adequate protein, vitamins, minerals and anti-oxidants.

3. **Chemicals in the food supply**:
   Fertilizers, pesticides and additives. Over 10,000 food and chemical additives are permitted in our food. The average American eats about 14 pounds of additives a year.

4. **Water contamination**:
   Water samples from cities across the US have been found to contain industrial chemicals, solvents, insect repellent, fire retardant, antibiotics, hormones, chemotherapy drugs and many other prescription and non-prescription drugs.

5. Air Pollution:

Besides such obvious offenders as autos and factories, we face the new danger of off-gassing from building and consumer products. Indoor air is found to contain benzene, styrene, carbon tetrachloride, formaldehyde and toluene from fabrics, furniture, curtains, carpet, padding, glues and plastics.

6. Dental Fillings:

Mercury may leach into the body in amounts high enough to cause health problems.

Consequences of not removing toxins:

- Chronic degenerative diseases. These include: arthritis, cancer, diabetes, heart disease, allergies, kidney failure, asthma, and digestive problems.

- Fatigue, irritability, muscle cramps, tremors, weakness and sleep disturbances.

- Hormonal disruption: This contributes to fibroids, PMS, infertility, female and male cancers and endometriosis.

- Suppressed immune function: Increased susceptibility to infections, colds, pneumonia, asthma, and flu.

- Chemical hypersensitivity, allergies and fibromylagia.

- Nervous system imbalances: Poor memory, mood disorders, depression, attention deficit disorders, hyperactivity, mental confusion, anxiety, and dementia.

- Headache, blurred vision, seizures, and dizziness.

- Digestive problems: Diarrhea, nausea, vomiting, loss of appetite and pain.

- Urinary frequency, recurrent infections and incontinence.

- Asthma and respiratory disorders.

- Skin irritation, and dermatitis.

- Joint and muscle pain.

- High blood pressure, and increased heart rate.

- Higher rates of cancer.

- Garlic breath (Arsenic), Yellow teeth (Cadmium).

Detoxification Summary

We live in a toxic world. Human testing shows that all of us have some detectable level of potentially toxic chemicals and metals. Scientific treatments consist of preventing exposure, removing the toxins and replenishing nutrients used for detoxification. This can be done safely and effectively during your **PWL** program.

7. Rejuvenation: Maximizing your nutritional potential

Rejuvenation means supercharging your body with the vitamins, minerals and other food factors that lead to optimum health and weight. Your cells are powerful little engines that make organs function (brain, liver, kidneys, muscles, bone, glands, etc). By providing higher levels of nutrients, your cells are better able to repair and rejuvenate themselves.

Studies show that the "average" person is deficient in at least three nutrients. These deficiencies won't kill you, but they will reduce the quality of your life and ability to maintain a healthy weight.

Sad to say, eating a "good diet" is no longer enough to supply us with all the nutrients we need. This is because our foods contain 30-50% fewer vitamins and minerals than they did fifty years ago. These figures are from the United States Department of Agriculture, not exactly a radical organization. Yes, you're trying to maintain health in an increasingly toxic world on a deficient diet. Fat chance, if you'll pardon the pun.

Simply put, when you don't have the nutrients you don't function as efficiently. It's like running your car on watered down gasoline. It might sputter along, but putting your pedal to the floor only causes a rougher ride. It's not very satisfying. That's how your life and weight will be as long as you're running on watered-down nutrition.

Another way to think about this is that for millions of years your ancestors ate pure, organic, nutrient-dense, unprocessed foods. There was no fast-food cheating because there were no fast foods. Then, in a relatively short period of time, just a hundred and fifty years, our diets switched to artificially grown, pesticide-laden, overly-processed, calorie-rich, nutrient-poor, standard American diets (SAD).

Are you deficient?

Just like with toxins, it's not a matter of if, but how deficient. Our goal at *PWC* is to determine which deficiencies are contributing to your health problems, including weight gain.

Unfortunately, the state of science at this time does not allow for easy nutritional testing. Vitamin D, for instance, is determined accurately by a blood test, but most standard blood tests for vitamins and minerals aren't particularly useful. The reason for this is that the blood tends to "steal" what it needs from tissues. For instance, the person with osteoporosis (loss of bone calcium) will usually have normal blood levels of calcium because the blood is "stealing" calcium from the bones.

Determining nutritional status

Since standard blood tests are only partially helpful, determining the state of your nutrition requires a more complex approach. Nutritionally-educated health practitioners look at your health history, do a thorough physical exam, and assess your laboratory results to come up with a comprehensive assessment of your nutritional status. While no one test proves a deficiency, weighing all these factors can lead to a successful treatment plan.

Health History

Valuable clues as to a person's nutritional status may come from their health history. For example, osteoporosis may indicate a calcium, phosphorus, magnesium, vitamin D or K deficiency. Eczema suggests essential fatty acid or zinc deficiencies (as well as trouble with fat absorption or allergies). Joint pain, especially with a family history of arthritis, may mean an omega-3 fatty acid deficiency. Low thyroid function may indicate a need for iodine, tyrosine, or vitamin D. Diabetics often need B-vitamins, chromium, and zinc.

Physical Exam

Essential fatty acid deficiencies often show up as dry skin. Thin nails may mean a calcium deficiency. A drop in standing blood pressure may indicate adrenal fatigue. Noisy joints or arthritic joints increase suspicion of a chondroitin problem. Loss of height with age often indicates osteoporosis. A zinc taste test can suggest that a person is low in zinc.

Laboratory testing

While not perfect, standard blood and urine tests for vitamins and minerals are of some help. As discussed elsewhere, a simple Free-Radical test (We do this test with all our patients.) can indirectly indicate the level of antioxidants (although there are many complicating factors). There is also an oral vitamin C test that can be helpful.

For those wishing to know more, a number of independent labs now offer **advanced testing** for nutrients. Generally these are expensive, in the range of a couple of hundred dollars, and not accepted by the medical establishment (Note that vitamin D testing, which is now becoming routine, was not accepted for many years.) At *Pure Wellness Centers* we often recommend a urine test for metabolic chemicals that indirectly indicates levels of B-vitamins, Co-Enzyme Q10 (important for cell energy generation), and glutathione (a powerful antioxidant).

The **PWL** program is not intended to diagnose or treat specific nutritional deficiencies. The diet, shakes, and supplements are loaded with high levels of rejuvenating nutrients. If you would like additional guidance on nutritional deficiencies, your **PW** doctor would be happy to see you for an individual consultation. These are usually paid for by insurance. Advanced testing is often recommended for those who are unable to lose weight on the **PWL** program.

The solution to nutritional deficiencies

There are two ways to correct nutritional deficiencies and rejuvenate cells.

- Eating nutrient-dense foods as opposed to the toxin-laden, nutrient-poor foods that make up most people's diets.

- Supplementing vitamins, minerals, and the other food factors necessary for rejuvenating cells.

The *Pure Weight Loss* program does both. As you read chapter 12, you'll see that an optimal (and tasty!) diet is described and nutritional supplements recommended. In addition, the **PWL** shake provides the nutrient density of several average meals.

Section III

Getting Started

"It's not a question of IF you're toxic, but how toxic you are."

Tom Ballard, ND

8. Information Gathering

A. Biomarkers: Before starting this program several **biomarkers** of health will be recorded. In addition to your weight, we also measure your **percentage of fat, water and muscle, your body-mass index (BMI) and take your body measurements.** With this information we can monitor your success at losing fat while retaining muscle.

Did you know that your **percentage of fat and your waist-to-hip ratio** are the best predictors of health? Statistics show that the higher these numbers are, the greater the chances are of cancer, diabetes, heart disease, and early death. These are important measurements that everyone should know.

B: Free Radicals: We will also be measuring your **free radical** levels. Free radicals are breakdown products from oxygen that damage healthy tissue. Outside your body, free-radicals cause fats to go rancid. Inside the body, free-radicals destroy cells, triggering inflammatory reactions. Overweight people tend to be highly inflamed; leading to pain, diabetes, heart disease, depression, and other chronic diseases.

C. Comprehensive Health History: You will be asked to fill out a detailed **health history**. Medical conditions such as low thyroid, digestive problems, hormone imbalances, chronic pain, and allergies may contribute to weight gain. While this program is not designed to address these problems, your **Pure Wellness** doctor will be happy to point out health issues that may be holding you back from your weight goals. At your request, we can address these issues in a separate visit or provide a referral to another qualified health professional.

D. Diet History: We also ask you to fill out a questionnaire about your **current diet**. Unfortunately, this vital information is missing from most health assessments. We can often point out areas of improvement that may tip the balance toward weight loss.

9. Advanced Testing

We highly recommend that you complete additional, advanced testing for toxins that may be compromising your health and weight loss. Toxin testing on ordinary people all over the planet has shown that everyone retains some degree of contaminants. The advantage of testing is that therapies can be made more specific. Different chemicals require different treatments.

- ## Toxic metal testing
  - o High levels of toxic metals are common, even in those without job exposure. For instance, tuna and metal dental fillings can increase mercury levels.
  - o We offer a home urine test for detecting high levels of toxic metals including lead, mercury, arsenic, aluminum, cadmium, and several others.
  - o Ask your doctor for a test kit that you can take home for this test.

- ## Environmental Toxin Testing
  - o Research studies indicate that virtually everyone holds toxins in their body; it's a question of which kind and how much.
  - o We offer a home urine test for 38 chemical markers for antioxidants, B-vitamins, solvents, pesticides, and other synthetic chemicals
  - o Ask your doctor for a test kit that you can take home for this test.

- ## Other Testing
  - o Because this program is designed to focus on weight-loss only, testing for other health

problems will not be recommended unless you are unable to lose weight on the basic program.

○ If you have health problems that you feel are holding you back from losing weight, we suggest that you make an appointment with your *PW* physician for a medical consultation. It could be that an important component of your health such as anemia, low thyroid, diabetes, or deficient vitamin B12 is preventing you from achieving a healthy weight. Generally, medical consultations are paid for by insurance. Check with your insurance provider.

Section IV

Your Pure Weight Loss

"One of the best things you can do to lose weight is to forget much of what you believe to be true about dieting, especially cutting calories and reducing fat. Before eliminating anything, ADD nutrient-rich, toxin-free foods."

Tom Ballard, ND

10.What to expect during your *Pure Weight Loss*

Healthy detoxification feels good. Yes, patients generally feel **energized, focused, and less stressed**.

You may have heard that detoxing, while good for you, feels terrible. This is wrong. When done right, you'll be surprised how much better you feel.

It is true that poorly-designed, nutrient-poor detox programs often leave you feeling weak, irritable, and with symptoms such as headaches and rashes. These are signs that you are not eliminating toxins, merely recycling them.

Remember, **toxins tend to be held in fat cells**. One of the goals of your detox is to **break down fat cells**, releasing the toxins. The toxins then travel to the liver where they are eliminated – if the liver is well nourished. That's the magic of the **PWL** program. Our **PW Shakes** provide you with the liver-supportive vitamins, minerals, antioxidants, and other nutrients necessary for efficient removal of toxins.

We caution patients that if they feel bad during their detox they should temporarily discontinue it and talk to us about modifying their program. This rarely happens, but is possible with highly toxic people.

Weight

Your body weight, and especially fat, will go down during your **PWL** program. However, it's important to remember that **our bodies cannot lose more than two to three pounds of fat per week**. This means you must be realistic and patient. If your goal is to lose 30 pounds then it will take 10 to 15 weeks to lose that much. Yes, it can be frustrating, but be assured that as you lose that weight you will become healthier. **A**

healthier you means a healthier weight which will be easier to maintain.

Fad diets that encourage loss of **5-10 pounds per week** ultimately lead to weight gain because they cause the loss of protein and water while turning down energy. This is a recipe for future weight gain, lethargy, and other metabolic and hormonal problems.

Energy
Most patients feel an increase in overall energy and sense of well being. With higher energy comes more calorie burning. Also look for an improvement in your stamina and a reduction in energy highs and lows.

Mood
Toxins and nutritional deficiencies tend to reduce energy. This is often reflected in the brain with depression, anxiety, insomnia and other neurological problems. Detoxification often lifts moods as it lightens toxin loads.

Digestion
The **PWL** program improves digestive function and elimination. Some patients may experience a temporary state of increased gas and bloating for a few days due to the increased fiber intake. This can be relieved by insuring that you have two or more bowel movements each day. Constipation is usually not a problem, but if it is, add 2-4 ounces of prune juice or more rice fiber to your shake. If constipation has been a chronic problem, make an appointment with your *Pure Wellness* doctor for a consultation.

Tell your doctor

It's important that you tell your doctor if you experience any unpleasant symptoms during your detoxification. Feeling bad can mean you have an unusually high level of toxins that aren't being removed efficiently.

Call or email your doctor so we can change your program so that you're eliminating toxins at a rate your body can handle. Not feeling well is an indication that more testing may be necessary to determine your toxic load.

11. Components of *Pure Weight Loss*

- **Attitude**: You are losing weight to become healthier so that you can live a fuller life for yourself, your friends and family. You know your goals will take time and effort, but will lead to rich rewards.

- **Meals**: Since nutritional deficiencies keep you from losing weight, you will be eating a healthy, balanced diet. Feeding yourself nutrient-dense foods increases energy and reduces appetite – both are essential for achieving a healthy weight.

- *Pure Wellness* **Meal Shakes**: These are a combination of specific vitamins, minerals, antioxidants, and other nutrients for detoxification and rejuvenation. Removing toxins increases the functioning of your hormones, nerves, and metabolism. Replacing missing nutrients boosts energy and fat-burning efficiency.

- **Activity**: Your body was created to move. Movement is part of life. Activity is fundamental to achieving your weight and health goals. While some people enjoy going to a gym, others prefer to incorporate activity into their life. Either strategy can work to help you lose weight. Remember, when you move you break down fat cells.

- **Mind/Body Detoxification Treatments:** A relaxing and detoxifying combination of massage, far-infrared heat, and serotonin enhancement available exclusively at *Pure Wellness Centers.*

- **Supplements**: Specific vitamins, minerals, antioxidants and other nutritional factors will boost fat burning and aid in your recovery from chronic weight problems.

- **Doctor Supervision and Monitoring:** We guide you to insure your success and avoid side effects. Your PW doctor will be your weight-loss partner.

12. Your Pure Weight Loss Program

A. Your Nutritious Eating Guide

Healthy eating is easy and delicious. It's not as complicated or unpleasant as you've been led to believe. The goal is to maximize the nutrients in your diet – thus turning your hunger off and your energy on. Below is a synthesis of the proven, core principles of healthy nutrition based on the historic record and sound nutritional research. (To find out more, read my book, *Nutrition-1-2-3: Three proven diet wisdoms for losing weight, gaining energy, and reversing chronic disease*)

Nutrition-1-2-3
Three proven diet wisdoms for gaining energy, losing weight, and reversing chronic disease.

Are all fats bad? Is high protein good? What about Dr. McFad's weight-loss program? Is it true carrots cause cancer? Experts argue. News reports confound. The food pyramid has collapsed. Should you give up?

Overwhelming scientific evidence proves that good nutrition is the most effective defense against obesity, diabetes, heart disease, cancer, arthritis and all other chronic diseases. Yet most people are baffled about how to shop and what to eat.

Nutrition, however, does not have to be so bewildering. Modern science actually supports ancient traditions. Healthy nutrition can be synthesized into three simple principles or Wisdoms for saving your life – **Regularity, Variety and Wholeness**.

1. **Regularity**: The regular intake (no skipping meals!) of food by hunter-gatherers is supported by current research in heart disease, diabetes, and obesity. This wisdom can change you from an overweight slug to a lean, vital person by increasing metabolism and blocking food cravings.

2. **Variety**: Unlike the current average intake of 20 foods, our ancestors ate hundreds. Research supports the health advantages of a mixed diet. One benefit: decreased appetite.

3. **Wholeness**: Science confirms the value of our ancestors' intake of fresh, un-processed, organic foods. Greater nutritional value translates into increased energy and reduced appetite.

The Three Wisdoms distil the essence of nutrition into a highly functional mantra: **Regularly eat a variety of whole foods.** This forms a powerful reference that applies to shopping, cooking, snacking, and eating out. It also provides a scientific basis for separating sound health claims from hype and fads.

To read more details on basic healthy nutrition see my book, ***Nutrition-1-2-3: Three diet wisdoms for losing weight, gaining energy, and reversing chronic disease.***

Twenty diet principles for healthy weight loss:

1. Your shopping and eating mantra: **Regularly eat a Variety of Whole foods.** (For details, see Chapter 14, or my book, ***Nutrition-1-2-3: Three diet wisdoms for losing weight, gaining energy, and reversing chronic disease***)

2. To provide maximum nutritional value, concentrate on **whole, organic, low-processed foods**. Avoid packaged foods which are low in nutrition and high in toxins.

3. All foods are to be **fresh, frozen, or dried**. No canned – the heat of canning reduces nutrients and the plastic lining adds a powerful hormone-disrupting toxin.

4. Never let yourself become extremely **hungry**. This indicates you're going too long between meals or not eating sufficient nutrients. Lack of nutrients = slowed fat burning.

5. Eat **breakfast, lunch, dinner** and at least **two small snacks** (mid-morning/mid-afternoon). The size should be kept small so - no overeating until stuffed. A constant intake of fuel keeps the metabolic fire burning.

6. **Snacks**: Eat at least two snacks a day, usually mid-morning and mid-afternoon. Snacks should always contain some form of protein. (No fruit alone, always pair with a protein such as nuts.) The **PW Shake** can be used as a snack.

7. Eat one handful of non-salted **tree nuts** two times daily (not peanuts). With fruit, carrot or celery they make a great snack.

8. Drink 8-10 cups of purified **water** daily to improve cellular efficiency. Start with 2 glasses on rising. Drink the majority before 3 pm. If you have bladder problems, work up to this over two weeks by adding ½ cup per day. During your appointments, we will be monitoring your hydration.

9. Eat **3 servings of vegetables and 2 servings of fruit** each day. A serving is ½ cup. Fresh, frozen, and low-heat dehydrated only, no canned.

10. For cooking use **organic extra-virgin olive oil or coconut oil**.

11. Salad dressings are best made with **organic extra-virgin olive oil.**

12. Cook with **low heat or a slow cooker** (crockpot). No microwave.

13. **Avoid sugar and sweetened** foods, both natural and artificial sources. Sugar is a highly processed, unnatural substance, that is more of a drug than a food. **Stevia, Lo Han (magic fruit), xylose and xylitol** are acceptable substitutions.

14. **Treats**: Sweets are a part of the celebration of life. Make them special, not a daily indulgence. Think of ways other than food to reward yourself. In choosing a treat, look for high quality and as close to natural as you can. Exotic fruits and homemade, natural treats are wonderful rewards.

15. **Never eat sweets or simple carbs alone**. When eating anything sweet, even fruits, always do so with or after a protein meal or snack. This slows the release of the sugar and its conversion into fat.

16. You'll be eating plenty of carbs in the form of vegetables and fruit, therefore eat **grains sparingly and preferably no wheat** (bread, muffins, wheat pasta, cookies, crackers). Wheat is highly addictive for some people making it difficult to lose weight.

17. **Avoid "low fat"** and "reduced fat" foods. These are processed foods. Good fats, as found naturally in nuts, seeds, avocados and whole dairy, help turn off your hunger center.

18. **Protein**: Eat ½ gram of protein per pound of body weight daily. (See page 45 - Protein content of common foods) If you weigh 150 pounds, that's 75 grams of protein a day. Every meal or snack should contain protein. Yes – even snacks are better with protein. Your **PW Shake** contains 26 grams of protein.

19. **No eating two hours before bedtime**, unless otherwise advised by your physician.

20. *Focus on the taste of what you <u>are</u> eating, instead of what you're not eating.*

Meal Planning

The number one rule of your eating day is to not become excessively hungry. Eating regular snacks, meals and shakes throughout the day stabilizes your blood sugar and harnesses your appetite resulting in weight loss.

The **PWL** shakes are filling. They may even be sufficient as a meal replacement. On the other hand, your metabolic needs may require you to supplement your shakes with other foods. That's not a problem. Eat. **Do not go hungry**. Going hungry will only lead to overeating and poor discipline.

Breakfast Ideas
- Generally the **PWL** *Shake* will be satisfying on its own and is ten times more nutritious than most meals.
- If the **PWL** *Shake* is not filling you may eat any other nutritious food you desire. For instance:
  - Oatmeal (steel cut, not instant)
  - Wheat-free cereal
  - Gluten-free toast
  - Fresh fruit
  - Nuts and seeds
  - Balanced nutrition bar (protein, carbs, fats)
  - Eggs (poached or hard-boiled, not fried)
  - Organic breakfast meats
  - Smoked salmon

Snack Ideas
- Nuts and seeds
- Fruits
- Nut butter (almond, cashew, sesame, filbert, etc. on apple or pear slices)
- Balanced nutrition bar
- Celery with nut butter
- Carrots, radishes, and other fresh vegetables

- Hummus with fresh vegetables
- Smoked salmon
- Hard-boiled egg

Lunch Ideas
- Steamed, grilled, or stir-fried mixed vegetables with a protein source such as chicken, beef strips, cheese, or hard-boiled egg
- Sandwich made from wheat-free bread
- Mixed green salad with a protein source such as chicken, beef strips, cheese
- Waldorf salad with smoked salmon for protein.
- Potato sandwich: Baked potato or yam sliced in half and used like bread to make a sandwich using lettuce, sprouts, cheese or other protein source
- Vegetable/protein soup (not from cans)
- Dinner leftovers

Dinner Ideas
- Steamed, grilled or stir-fried vegetables
- Baked, grilled or poached fish
- Same foods you eat for lunch
- Quiche with vegetables
- Homemade baked casseroles (great for leftovers)
- Lasagna with wheat-free noodles
- Baked squash and baked chicken with a salad.
- Spaghetti squash instead of wheat spaghetti with pesto sauce and beef cubes.
- Make enough for tomorrow's lunch

Common dietary mistakes leading to weight gain

- Consuming low-nutrient foods – high in calories, low in vitamins, minerals, and other nutrients.
- Not eating a protein-rich breakfast.
- Eating late in the evening.
- Eating too fast without adequate chewing.
- Missing meals.
- Eating excessively large meals.

First Choice/Last Choice Reminder

First Choice	Last Choice
Whole unprocessed foods	Processed, degraded
Fresh, frozen, dried	Cans, boxes, packages
Organic	Non-organic
Extra virgin olive and coconut oil	Soy and corn oil
Unsweetened,or	Sugar, fructose, corn sweetener
stevia,LoHan,xylose, or xylitol.	Skipping meals
Regular meals and snacks	Wheat
Quinoa, millet, amaranth, rice	Tap and water in soft plastic
Filtered water	Grain fed
Free-range, organic meat	Fast food
Home cooked	Cola, fruit juice, sugared drinks
Water	Coffee
Green Tea (organic)	Gulping
Chewing	

Most likely contaminated with pesticides
- Peaches
- Apples and pears
- Imported grapes
- Spinach
- Potatoes

Least likely contaminated with pesticides
- Onions
- Avocado
- Pineapple and mango
- Frozen sweet peas and corn
- Asparagus
- Kiwi
- Bananas
- Cabbage and broccoli
- Eggplant

www.foodnews.org has a handy shopper's guide

B. *Pure Wellness* Meal Shakes

This delicious shake is a complete meal replacement and detoxification formula containing 26 grams of protein, 7 grams of fiber, and 3 mg of medium chain triglycerides (good fats), plus a unique combination of vitamins, minerals, amino acids, antioxidants and herbs for restoring maximum vitality. It is packed with nutrients – several times more than most meals.

Your shake is food, not a supplement. It is more nutritious than most meals. Just because it comes dehydrated and powdered, does not make it "not real food". People have been dehydrating foods for thousands of years. While it is delicious, nutritious and filling, you're encouraged to also eat other foods, meals, and snacks with an emphasis on organic fruits and vegetables.

The basic shake is made with:

- Pure water: 8-10 ounces.
- ProtoClear: One (1) scoop.
- Stabilized Rice Fiber: Four (4) tablespoons.
- MCT oil: 3/4 tablespoon.

(Chapter 20 contains more shake recipes.)

Ingredient Details

- **ProtoClear**: one (1) scoop
    - Hypoallergenic: no wheat, dairy, soy, corn, or eggs.
    - Rice and pea protein based.
    - Added nutrients to aid detoxification and replenish deficient nutrients.
    - 22 grams of protein per scoop.
    - Medium chain triglycerides for energy and weight loss.

- o No added sugars, preservatives, artificial sweeteners.
- o Good Manufacturing Processes (GMP) certified.
- o Mixes easily without a blender.
- o Tastes great.

- **Stabilized Rice Bran Fiber**: 4 tablespoons
  A natural combination of:
  - o A non-irritating rice bran fiber used for centuries. for its nutrient content.
  - o Stabilized to prevent rancidity.
  - o Natural antioxidants.
  - o Mixes easily in water.
  - o A delicious, slightly nutty flavor.

- **MCT Oil**: 3/4 tablespoon
  - o MCT = Medium chain triglycerides.
  - o An extract from healthy coconut oil..
  - o Stimulates metabolism and weight loss.
  - o Suppresses appetite.
  - o Mild flavor.
  - o Read more in chapter 18 on coconut oil.

Mixing your shake
Add water and shake ingredients in a container with a tight lid and shake to mix, or place ingredients in a blender and blend. Adding ice to the blender makes for a smoother drink. We recommend the basic ingredients with water, however fresh or frozen fruit may also be added. See chapter 20 of this book for more mixing ideas.

Eat your shake
Your shake is a meal or part of a meal. As with all foods, avoid gulping or chugging your shake. For maximum digestibility, sip it over 10 to 20 minutes.

Timing your shakes

- **Days 1-4: Introduction**
  - Introduce your *Pure Weight Loss Shake* slowly by using the **ProtoClear** portion of the shake only. Mix one-half (1/2) scoop ProtoClear in 4-8 ounces of water. Drink this within 45 minutes of waking.

- **Days 5-21: Induction** (until end of third week)
  - Drink the **full Pure Weight Loss Shake** (ProtoClear, Rice Fiber, & MCT Oil) within 45 minutes of waking.
    - Increases your energy
    - Increases your fat burning
    - Increases your detoxification
    - Reduces your appetite

- **Day 22-42: Intensive** (until end of six weeks)
  - Continue your full morning shake
  - **Add a second shake** around 3pm, or 2-3 hours before dinner.
    - Gives you an afternoon boost of energy and mental alertness
    - Reduces your appetite for the most fattening meal of the day, dinner.
    - You will find that your dinners will become smaller and more enjoyable.

Pure Weight Loss Shake Recipes

Start with the basic shake, and then improvise as desired for taste.

Basic Shake:
- Pure Water: 8-12 ounces
- ProtoClear (Vanilla, Berry, or Orange): One scoop
- MCT Oil : 3/4 Tbsp
- Rice Fiber: 4 Tbsp
- Shake or blend ingredients

Variations:
- Substitute rice or nut milk for water (Note: this adds calories.)
- Add ice when blending; this creates a smoother shake.
- Substitute coconut, rice or almond milk for ¼ - ½ water.
- Blend with fresh or frozen fruit.
- If you find the shake too sweet, add fresh lemon.
- Substitute fruit juice for the water. (This will be too sweet for most people.)

Pina Colada
- Substitute coconut and pineapple juice for water.
- 1 scoop vanilla ProtoClear
- MCT Oil: 3/4 Tbsp
- Rice Fiber: 4 Tbsp.
- Blend with ice.

Apple-Lemon Ginger Snap
- Substitute one half of water with apple juice.
- 1 scoop berry ProtoClear
- MCT Oil: 3/4 Tbsp
- Rice Fiber: 4 Tbsp
- 1-2 oz of fresh lemon juice

- 1 Tbsp of ginger juice
- Blend with water and/or ice

Tropical Breeze
- 2 oz of coconut milk.
- 1 scoop berry or orange ProtoClear
- MCT Oil: 3/4 Tbsp
- Rice Fiber: 4 Tbsp
- 4 oz of water
- 1/4 cup papaya/mango or banana.
- Blend with or without ice.

Berry Delightful
- 1 scoop berry ProtoClear
- MCT Oil: 3/4 Tbs.
- Rice Fiber: 4 Tbs.
- 1 cup of fresh or frozen berries
- 8 oz of cold water or rice milk

Berry Tart
- 1 scoop Berry ProtoClear
- MCT Oil: 3/4 Tbsp
- Rice Fiber: 4 Tbsp
- 4 oz of pomegranate juice
- 2 oz of unsweetened cranberry juice

V-48
- 1 scoop orange ProtoClear
- MCT Oil: 3/4 Tbsp
- Rice Fiber: 4 Tbsp
- 4-6 oz of carrot or mixed vegetable juice or one scoop GreensFirst
- 4-6 oz of water

Minty Orange
- 1 scoop of orange ProtoClear

- MCT Oil: 3/4 Tbsp
- Substitute cold mint tea for water or one scoop GreensFirst (which contains mint). This may also be served warm.

* Fiber quantities may be reduced for a smoother taste. Blending with ice also makes for a smoother shake.

C. Activity: Movement, standing, walking, hustle, bustle, and exercise

Life does not exist without activity. It comes in many levels, from toe twitching to tap dancing. Activity is a less scary and more inclusive word than exercise. If you're already exercising regularly, keep it up. If you hate the thought of exercise, add more fun activities to your life.

- Aim for a minimum of **60 minutes 4 times a week** in which your heart rate is over 100.

- Choose something you **enjoy** doing or can do with friends. Some people find that music or books on tape helps to keep them going.

- If you walk the dog, **keep moving** to increase your heart rate – it's good for both of you.

- If you drive, **park your car twice as far** away from your destination as you would usually.

- If you've been taking the elevator, remember the scene from *The Silence of the Lambs* and **take the stairs**.

- Meet friends and colleagues for a **walk instead of coffee**.

- **Rebounders, jump ropes, weighted hoops** (a hoola hoop with weight inside) and **Soloflex whole-body vibration** are excellent ways to exercise.

- While watching TV or otherwise sedentary pastimes, add **stretching and other activities**. Push ups or yoga during commercials? Leg extensions while sitting on the couch?

- Remember **isometrics**? Push your hands and knees together while sitting in your office chair. Press on an immovable object, like the roof of your car, while at a red light (While stopped!).

- Garage, yard sales, and thrift stores have great bargains on **exercise equipment**. Set them up in your TV room.

- **Avoid sitting** for more than two hours. After that hormones kick in that cause muscle loss and fat gain. Even a few minutes of standing or walking reverses this negative trend. It will also increase your circulation and renew your mental focus.

- Your success will increase as you learn to incorporate activities you enjoy into your daily life.

D. Mind/Body Detoxification treatments

Detoxification is integral to health. Every cell in your body relies on taking in nutrients and removing waste. Detoxing helps with weight loss by improving the energy and efficiency of cells.

Detoxification has been practiced by every civilization throughout history. Saunas, mud baths, herb wraps, mineral springs, and sweat lodges are examples of how our ancestors helped keep themselves healthy.

Doctors at **Pure Wellness Centers** have developed a detoxification method that adapts ancient practices to modern lifestyles. We call it **Pure Mind/Body Detoxification** (MBD). This therapy safely and pleasantly increases detoxification, calms the central nervous system, and increases healing serotonin. Stress, anxiety, and sleep problems add to your toxic load and make it difficult to lose weight.

The therapy

During a MBD treatment you will be lying on your back on a table containing 32 heated rollers. You will be fully clothed, preferably in loose natural-fiber clothing. The rollers are **controlled by a computer** and will adjust to your body as they roll up and down the muscles and **acupuncture points** along your spine.

Far-infrared heat, the same heat the sun generates, will heat your body from below and above. **This combination of massage and acupressure is very pleasant and often helps patients with back pain and sciatica.**

While you are relaxing with the heat and massage you will be feeling the pleasing effects of **Cranial Electrotherapy**

Stimulation (CES). CES sounds other-worldly, but is simply microcurrent therapy. It is safe, approved by the FDA, and has over 50 years of research support. The unit is clipped to your earlobes. CES has been shown to increase relaxing alpha waves and serotonin levels.

Serotonin helps clear **depression**, improves **sleep**, reduces **carb cravings**, and lessens **pain** and **anxiety**. Patients often find their mood lifts, they sleep improves, and they are **calmer under stress**.

As part of your *Pure Weight Loss* program we recommend at least one 30 minute MBD treatment each week. Five 60 minute sessions are included in the price of this program. Arrangements can be made for more treatments for a small additional fee.

Other detoxification strategies

Health involves continuous detoxification to remove waste products and environmental toxins. When our patients are not able to utilize our Mind/Body Detoxification we recommend:

- Physical activities that increase sweating
- Far-Infrared sauna
- Epsom Salt baths (4-6 cups in hot bath for 30 minutes)
- Skin brushing (sponges and brushes are available for removing dead skin and promoting circulation)
- Mud and herbal wraps
- Hot teas that induce sweating
- Massage
- Yoga and stretching

E. *Pure Wellness* Supplements

Along with your **Pure Weight Loss Shake** there are additional supplements to help you lose weight by increasing detoxification pathways and maximizing nutritional rejuvenation. We ask that you use only **Pure Wellness** supplements because they are of the very highest quality and purity. If you are already taking another brand of supplements, please set them aside for now. You may reintroduce them later, after your health has improved.

- **Niacin**
  Niacin mobilizes fat cells. This increases fat loss and removal of toxins that are held in fat cells. Niacin has been used successfully in treating toxins involved in Gulf War Syndrome and with rescue workers contaminated during the 9/11 disaster.

  Dosage: Take one (1) capsule with your morning shake unless otherwise advised by your physician.

- **ChromeMate®** (chromium complex)
  ChromeMate® contains a unique patented niacin-bound chromium complex. Chromium is an essential trace mineral that works with insulin to support healthy blood glucose levels already within the normal range and plays an important role in the proper utilization of protein, fat and carbohydrates. Independent studies show that ChromeMate® provides greater biological activity than other chromium supplements tested. By stabilizing blood sugar, it reduces sweet cravings.

  Dosage: Take one (1) capsule twice daily with your morning shake and evening meal unless otherwise advised by your physician.

Additional Supplements

Your **PW** physician may decide that your condition requires additional nutrients. This may be because your body needs higher levels either to encourage healthy detoxification or to replace deficient nutrients.

Common examples are:

- **Special-2 or True Balance Multivitamin**
  These formulas are high in stress-relieving B vitamins as well as vitamins A, C, D, E, and minerals in a digestible GMP approved tablet or capsule.

  Dosage: Take two (2) capsules with your morning shake unless otherwise advised by your physician.

- **Ultra Pure Omega Oil**
  These are highly concentrated omega-3 oil capsules (EPA 500/DHA 250) that help with weight loss by providing neurological support and reducing inflammation.

  Dosage: Take two (2) capsules twice daily with a shake or meals unless otherwise advised by your physician.

- **Calcium and Magnesium**
  These minerals are commonly deficient. They provide needed muscle and nerve support.

  Dosage: Take two (2) capsules with dinner unless otherwise advised by your physician.

- **GreensFirst or Red Alert**

  These are high-quality dehydrated organic fruit and vegetable drinks. They are helpful for patients with high levels of free radicals and showing signs of oxidative damage as in chronic inflammation. GreensFirst has more green vegetables. Red Alert is higher in berries. Both have the **antioxidant powers of more than 10 servings of fruits and vegetables**. They contain no grasses, added sugars, or artificial additives and are hypoallergenic.

  Dosage: One half to one scoop with water or added to the **PWL** shake.

- **Other supplements**

  While you may have heard of other supplements such as **carnitine, alpha-keto, hoodia and pyruvate**, we have not found them necessary when patients are supplied with sufficient nutrients and detoxified.

F. Program summary

The **PWL** program consists of:

- **Real Food**: Regularly eating a Variety of Whole foods.

- Nutritious detoxifying real food **shakes.**

- Daily **activity.**

- **Mind/Body detoxification treatments.**

- Detoxifying and rejuvenating **supplements.**

- Regular monitoring of **BioMarkers** by your **PWL** doctor to insure that you're losing fat, not muscle or water.

- Measurement of your **Free-Radicals** to monitor your detoxification progress.

This program will not interfere with your work or home life. It has been designed to take a minimal amount of time for maximum results.

13. Monitoring your weight loss

We recommend that you stay away from your home scale. Fixating on daily weight can be distracting. Remember, weight changes are due to water, muscle, and fat fluctuations. For most people the first sign of improvement in body composition is a change in how clothes fit.

Rather than your overall weight, concentrate on your food intake, activity, shakes, and supplements. The most important monitoring tool is your overall energy. As your energy increases, your fat will decrease.

Occasionally a patient's overall weight will not drop for the first several weeks. This may be because they were dehydrated or had poor muscle development. During the program their fat percentage went down, but their water and muscle percentages went up. Overall, this is good because being **well-hydrated and muscled can boost energy by as much as 15 percent**. After this initial period of gaining intercellular water (not edema) and muscle, your overall weight will begin dropping.

If this program is not helping you lose weight then we highly recommend that you consult with your **PW** naturopathic doctor about factors that may be interfering with your ability to lose fat. Anemia, thyroid, adrenal, B12 deficiency, and other metabolic problems can make it difficult to impossible to lose fat, even when eating well and exercising regularly.

Section VI

Supporting your weight loss

"You cannot rely on corporate food and media to support your healthy intentions. They have their goal – profits – and you have yours – vital health. Seek out others that share your goals. Be a revolutionary; eat, live, and think health for yourself and the planet."

Tom Ballard, ND

14. Protein Content of Common Foods
(In Grams)

Grains:
Amaranth: 1 cup, 28 grams
Bagel: 1, 9
Dinner roll: 1, 2.4
WW Bread: 1 slice, 2.4
English Muffin: 1, 4.5
Bran Flakes: 1 cup, 4.8
Oatmeal: 1 cup, 6
Sugar Frosted Flakes: 1 cup, 2
Rice Cake: 1, 0.7
Rye Crisp: 1 square, 6
Wheat thins: 8. 1.0
Brown rice: 1 cup, 14.5
Egg noodles: 1 cup, 6.6
Millet: 1 cup, 22.6
Quinoa: 1 cup, 22
Popcorn: 1 cup, 1.5
Spaghetti (WW) 1 cup, 8.4

Legumes:
Black Beans: 1 cup, 15
Garbanzo Beans: 1 cup, 14.5
Lentils: 1 cup, 18.0
Split Peas: 1 cup, 16
Soybeans: 1 cup, 28.6

Dairy:
Cheddar Cheese: 1 oz, 7.1
Cottage Cheese: 1 cup, 25
Feta Cheese: 1 oz, 4.0
Jack Cheese: 1 oz, 6.9
Whole Milk: 1 cup, 8.0
Yogurt -plain: 1 cup, 8
Yogurt - skim: 1 cup, 13
Egg: 1, 6.0

Misc:
Spirulina: 1 cup, 8.6
Tempeh: 100 gm, 19
Tofu, firm: 1/2c, 10

Meat:
Flank Steak: 4 oz, 22 grams
Lean Grd Beef: 4 oz, 28
Round Steak: 4 oz, 22
Lamb chop: 4 oz, 25.5
Bacon: 3 slices, 5.8
Ham: 3.5 oz, 18.5
Roll Chicken: 2 slices, 11
Chicken - drumstick: 1, 14
Chicken: 3.5 oz, 27
Turkey: 3.5 oz, 28
Turkey Roll: 2 slices, 10.3

Fish:
Cod: 3 oz, 19.4
Crab: 3 oz, 16.5
Halibut: 3 oz, 22.7
Oysters: 3 oz, 12
Salmon - pink: 3 oz, 16.8
Salmon - sockeye: 3 oz, 23.2
Shrimp: 3 oz, 17.8
Tuna in water: 1 can, 42

Nuts and Seeds:
Almonds: 1 oz, 4.6: 1 cup, 26.4
Almond Butter: 1 Tbs, 2.4
Cashews: 1 oz, 4.4: 1 cup, 24
Hazelnuts: 1 oz, 3.7
Pumpkin Seeds: 1 oz, 7.0: 1cup,40.6
Sunflower Seeds 1 oz 6.5: 1cup, 35
Sesame Butter (Tahini): 1 Tbs, 2.6
Walnuts: 1 oz, 4.1: 1 cup,14.8
Soy milk: 1 cup, 4-8

Vegetables:
Broccoli: ½ cup, 2.3
Carrot: ½ cup, 0.9
Baked Potato: 1 large, 4.7
Zucchini: ½ cup, 0.6

15. Tasty Detox Recipes
Adapted by Candace McNaughton, ND

Home Fries
Serves 4

- 8 small red potatoes
- 2 tsp olive or coconut oil
- 1 chopped onion
- ¼ tsp sea salt
- 1 tsp fresh rosemary, chopped
- Pepper to taste

Clean potatoes and cut into ¼ inch thick rounds. Steam for 7-10 minutes. Heat oil in skillet. Sauté onion until soft. Add potatoes and spices. Brown potatoes and serve hot.

Spicy Tempeh Stir-fry
Serves 4

- ¼ cup peanut oil
- ¼ cup tamari
- 8 oz tempeh, cubed
- ½ Tbsp olive oil or coconut oil
- ½ Tbsp sesame oil
- ½ small onion, sliced
- 1 Tbsp miso
- ¼ c vegetable stock
- 4 cup assorted vegetables, sliced
- 4 Tbsp tamari (wheat free)

Stir ¼ cup peanut oil and ¼ cup tamari together. Toss in tempeh. Bake 10 min at 425 degrees. In a large skillet, heat remaining oils. Add onion and cook for 2 min. Add remaining vegetables and cook for 2 more minutes. Add stock, tamari, cooked tempeh, and miso. Lower heat and simmer for 3-5 min.

Red Bean Chili
Serves 6
- 2 cups red beans
- 1 tsp cumin seeds
- 1 tsp dried oregano
- 2 Tbsp mild chili powder
- 2 bay leaves
- 1 onion, diced
- 1 clove garlic minced
- 2 cups chopped tomatoes
- 1 green pepper diced
- 1 Tbsp pureed chipotle peppers
- vinegar to taste

Rinse and soak the beans overnight. Pour off the water and put in fresh water to a couple of inches above the beans. Bring to a boil and skim off foam.

Or, use organic canned beans. Add the oregano, cumin, chili powder, onion and garlic. Cook over medium heat for 15 minutes. Add tomato, green pepper, and chipotle pepper. Simmer for 1 hour. Add vinegar just before serving to sharpen flavor.

Eggplant, Zucchini and Peppers Baked with Rice
This is delicious when made the day before and then reheated. It's also very good cold.
- ½ cup long-grain white or brown rice
- ½ cup olive oil
- 5 garlic cloves
- 4 medium-sized onions, sliced
- 1 medium-sized eggplant, peeled and cut into ½-inch cubes

- 3-4 medium-sized zucchini, sliced into 1/8" rounds
- 5-6 medium-sized red or green bell peppers, seeded, de-ribbed and cut into strips
- 9 medium-sized tomatoes, peeled, seeded and chopped, or (2) 35 oz. cans tomatoes drained
- 3 Tbsp chopped fresh parsley and basil leaves
- ½ cup chicken stock (wheat-free)
- salt and pepper to taste

Stir the rice into 2 quarts boiling salted water and cook for 8 minutes. Drain the rice and refresh it under cold running water. Set aside to drain thoroughly.

Heat oil in a 6-8 quart ovenproof casserole with lid. Add the garlic and onions and gently sauté them over medium-low heat for 6-8 minutes, stirring occasionally until the onions are clear and beginning to soften. Stir in the eggplant. After 2 minutes, stir in the zucchini and cook for 20 minutes, stirring frequently. Remove 2/3 of the vegetables from the casserole.

Spread the remaining vegetables in a layer and add alternating layers of red or green bell peppers, tomatoes, rice and cooked vegetables until all of the ingredients are used up, seasoning as you go with herbs. Sprinkle the top with herbs, pour on the chicken stock, cover the casserole and bake in a preheated 350 F oven for one hour. The vegetables should be very tender, but intact. Serves 8-10

Millet with Nuts and Raisins
- 1 cup millet
- 3 cups chicken stock (wheat-free)
- 1 large onion, chopped
- 2 Tbsp olive oil
- 1 tsp sea salt
- ¼ cup golden raisins

- 1 ounce pistachios or almonds, toasted and slivered (about ¼ cup)

Stirring constantly, toast the millet in an ungreased skillet over medium heat for 3-4 minutes, or until golden. Add all of the remaining ingredients except the nuts. Tightly cover the skillet, reduce the heat to low and simmer for 15 minutes or until millet is tender and the chicken stock is absorbed. Stir in the nuts and toss lightly. Correct the seasoning and serve warm. Serves 6

Persian Rice with Lentils and Chicken
- 1 ¼ cup long grain white or brown rice
- ¼ cup dried lentils
- ¼ cup dried apricots (sulfite-free), coarsely chopped
- 2 ounces almonds, blanched, sliced (about ½ cup) or use coarsely chopped pecans
- 2 Tbsp olive or coconut oil
- 1 medium onion, chopped
- 3 whole chicken breasts, boned, skinned and cut into ½-inch cubes
- 1 Tbsp finely chopped fresh dill

Soak the apricots in warm water for 30 minutes before cooking time, unless they are very soft. Sauté' nuts in oil until golden. Remove them from the pan and sauté the onions and chicken in the remaining oil, adding a little extra oil if necessary. Cook the onions until clear and soft and beginning to brown lightly. Remove chicken and onions from heat and set aside.

Bring 6 cups water to a boil, seasoning with salt. Add the lentils and cook for 5 minutes. Sprinkle in the rice and stir, allowing the water to boil again. Boil the rice and lentils for another 20 minutes, until they are just cooked. Have the chicken cubes at room temperature and apricots drained and squeezed out. Remove the rice-lentil mixture from the heat, drain in a colander, rinsing with very hot water.

Drain the mixture well and return it to the pot, mixing in the chicken and onions well so that the heat of the rice mixture heats the chicken through. Add apricots, sautéed nuts and dill. Toss gently and serve immediately. Serves 4-6

Borscht
This soup can be served hot or cold.
- 2 cups finely shredded cabbage
- 2 cups boiling water
- ½ cup chopped onion
- 2 Tbsp olive oil
- 1 pound cooked small beets, peeled, chopped (save the cooking water), as in the above recipe
- 1-quart chicken or vegetable stock (wheat-free)
- 2 tsp caraway seed
- 1 tsp honey, if desired
- 3 Tbsp. lemon juice
- salt and pepper to taste

Cook the cabbage for ten minutes in boiling, salted water. Cook the onion in the oil for a few minutes, without browning. Drain the beets, saving the cooking liquid, and chop them fine.

Add the chicken or vegetable stock to the onions. Upon boiling, add the cabbage and its cooking liquid. Add the beets, one cup of beet cooking liquid, caraway seeds, honey, salt and pepper to taste. Simmer for ten minutes, skimming carefully. Remove the soup from the heat. Add lemon juice and heat just to the boiling point. Serve with dill weed garnish.

Dr. Ballard's Waldorf Salad

This recipe adds protein and healthy fat to this traditional salad.

Serves 1 or two

- One diced apple
- 12 grapes
- Any other diced fruit you want to add (pear, mango, etc)
- One chopped celery stick
- Grated carrot (optional)
- ¼ cup organic mayonnaise or coconut milk
- A few pinches of cinnamon to taste
- ¼ cup diced smoked salmon

Toss and enjoy for breakfast, lunch, dinner or snack.

In preparing meals, challenge yourself to think outside the breadbox and your own culture. Experiment and enjoy!

16. Organic Virgin Coconut Oil

The Healthy Fat: Ignites weight loss, heads off heart disease, and restores youthful skin

Coconut oil has been used as a nutritious food and skin conditioner for thousands of years. Sadly, it fell out of favor in the 1960s when the food industry and MDs with no nutrition education started making false claims that it contains cholesterol and should be avoided. Yes, it is a saturated fat, but all saturated fats do not contain cholesterol. Cholesterol is only found in animal products. Saturated fats are, in fact, necessary for optimum health.

Back in the 1930's, Dr. Weston Price, a dentist, traveled throughout the South Pacific, examining traditional diets and their effect on dental and overall health. He found that **those eating diets high in coconut products were healthy and trim**, despite the high fat concentration in their diet.

Similarly, in 1981, researchers studied populations of two Polynesian atolls. Coconut was the chief source of caloric energy in both groups. The results, published in the *American Journal of Clinical Nutrition*, demonstrated that **heart and vascular disease was uncommon** in both populations. There was no evidence that the high saturated fat intake had a harmful effect in these populations.

Many other studies have confirmed the benefits of coconut oil.

Despite the evidence, the misinformation continues to this day. It is so pervasive that even people living in coconut-growing countries avoid this healthy food and instead use unhealthy vegetable oils. This has taken a toll on their health in the form of increasing rates of heart disease, diabetes, and obesity.

A few proven benefits of coconut oil:
- Supports weight loss.
- Improves athletic performance.
- Reduces risk of heart disease.
- Immune system support.
- Reduces cancer risk.
- A rapid energy source.
- Increases energy like carbohydrates, but does not cause wide fluctuations in blood sugar.
- Prevents and treats bacterial, viral and yeast infections
- Easily digested and assimilated.
- Protects skin from UV light damage and wrinkles.

Are your cooking oils killing you?

Despite the propaganda from the food industry, **corn, soy, safflower, sunflower and canola** oils are the **worst** oils for cooking. These polyunsaturated oils are very heat sensitive, breaking down and releasing damaging free radicals. Free radicals increase the incidence of cancer, Alzheimer's disease, diabetes, obesity, and degenerative disease in general. Saturated fats such as coconut oil are heat stable, making them ideal for cooking.

The Uniqueness of Coconut Oil

Coconut oil is comprised of medium-chain fatty acids (MCFAs), also called medium-chain triglycerides or MCTs. MCTs are healthy oils and coconut oil is the richest source. MCTs are smaller than most fats so pass into membranes without difficulty. They're also easy to digest and are converted quickly by the liver into energy rather than being stored as fat. **This quick energy stimulates metabolism and weight loss**.

Back in the 1940's, farmers discovered the stimulating effect of coconut oil by accident. They tried using the inexpensive coconut oil to fatten their livestock. It didn't work! Instead, their animals became lean, active and hungry. **Every farmer's nightmare is your dream come true!**

While coconut oil acts like carbohydrates in its ability to be "burned" for energy, it **does not require insulin** to be used by cells. This makes it an excellent choice for **diabetes, hypoglycemia**, and those with blood-sugar swings. In fact, the ability of MCFAs to be easily digested, and turned into energy has entered the sports arena. Several studies have shown that MCTs enhance physical and athletic performance.

The lauric acid found in coconuts has been shown to fight viruses, bacteria, yeast, fungi, and parasites. It can be used internally and locally on skin conditions.

Organic - Avoid processing and pesticides

Virgin coconut oil is made from fresh coconuts -- opened less than 48 hours after they are picked from the trees. These coconuts are grown and processed organically, without harmful fertilizers, additives or chemical solvents. Remember, pesticides and other harmful chemicals are stored in fat cells. This makes it especially important to choose organic when buying fat-rich foods such as coconut, avocados, eggs, dairy and meats.

Taste the value of coconut oil

Virgin coconut oil has a fresh, mild, light coconut flavor. It is non-greasy with no cholesterol and no trans-fats. Since it is solid at room temperature, it can be used like butter as a spread. Coconut oil is great for stir-fry or sauté, eggs, fish, and chicken. Add to your smoothie or juiced drinks for a delicate flavor and metabolic boost.

More than skin deep

Coconut oil is a favorite with professional massage therapists because of its skin-nourishing effect. It aids in removing the outer layer of dead skin cells, making the skin smoother. Coconut oil prevents formation of destructive free radicals that cause skin aging. This also protects the skin from sun damage and wrinkling. MCTs penetrate into the deeper layers of the skin to strengthen the underlying tissues. Recent research finds that healthy skin has a higher percentage of saturated fat over unsaturated fats. This means that coconut oil is better suited than poly-unsaturated oils such as safflower for use on the skin.

17. Food Allergies/Sensitivities and Weight

An allergy or sensitivity is a negative reaction to a food or environmental factor. Dust, pollens, and molds are well-known triggers. Certain foods can also cause reactions including weight gain.

Allergy or Sensitivity?

An allergic reaction occurs when the body produces an antibody (Ab) to a foreign protein (antigen). For instance, gluten, a protein in wheat and some other grains, may trigger an antibody reaction. In this case the person's immune system is "overly protective", mistaking gluten for a toxin in the person with allergies.

Sensitivities are reactions that do not involve foreign proteins and antibody production. The person may react to something such as sugar which contains no protein, yet it triggers a reaction such as a headache, mood change, or other unpleasant sensation.

Symptoms

Many people think allergic reactions only cause "hay fever" symptoms such as a runny nose or itching eyes. While these symptoms are common, many other reactions may occur. In fact, almost any part of the body may be affected.

- **Inflammation of any mucous membrane**
  Itching or mucous discharge of the eyes and nose occurs in mild cases. Headaches and sinus infections are the result of more severe reactions. Mucous

membranes of the **digestive** and **urinary** systems may also become involved. Bloating, gas, diarrhea, constipation and irritable bowel syndrome are common. Frequent urination, bed wetting and recurrent urinary-tract infections are also symptoms. Asthma and breathing problems may be triggered. It is worth investigating for allergies and sensitivities when a person has recurrent illness involving mucous membranes.

- **Irritation of serous membranes**
  Serous membranes line joints and allow for ease of movement. Allergies have been shown to trigger joint pain in some individuals.

- **Skin rashes**
  Eczema and other skin conditions are common among sensitive people.

- **Brain and Nervous System reactions**
  Food sensitivities occur often in patients with depression, learning disabilities, attention deficit disorder, agitation, poor concentration, mental cloudiness, and dyslexia. **Patients often crave and over eat foods they're sensitive to.** This is due to the release of endorphins that cause a temporary "high" feeling.

- **Energy**
  Fatigue, brain fog, and insomnia are common reactive symptoms. **Fatigue can lead to overeating,**

especially high caloric carbohydrates in an attempt to boost energy.

Note that the common thread in these conditions is **inflammation** and that the reaction may be delayed for up to 48 hours after ingesting the food.

Testing
Skin scratch tests are well-known to be inaccurate (Lawsuits have resulted from a patient being told they were allergy-free when they should have been warned that the test is only a guide and not reliable.)

Blood testing for antibodies (for instance, the RAST or ELISA tests for IgG or IgE) is only good for detecting true allergies but not sensitivities because they rely on detecting antibodies.

The **Food Elimination-Challenge**, although difficult to implement, is considered to be the most accurate way of detecting food allergies and sensitivities. See below for instructions.

Complicating factors
- It's possible to react to more than one food. Sometimes mild sensitivities to two or more foods trigger a more severe reaction. (Mild dairy + mild wheat = strong reaction to pizza. Or, living in a moldy house + corn allergy = daily fatigue with occasional headaches when eating corn).
- A food to which you are mildly sensitive may still cause a reaction if the food is eaten repeatedly. (For example:

Cream in coffee three times a day every day, even when no other dairy is eaten.)

Elimination-Challenge

- Step one: Decide which foods you want to test. There are three possibilities.
  - If you've ever noticed any foods bothering you, that's a good place to start.
  - If you have a craving for any foods, or find yourself eating the same foods every day, these are good candidates for testing. (Food sensitivities sometimes stimulate the release of endorphins which cause a craving for that food).
  - If you have no idea which foods you're reacting to, try the most commonly sensitive foods: **Wheat, oats, dairy*, soy, corn, eggs, peanuts, tomatoes, potatoes, and citrus fruit.**** These are the most commonly eaten foods, and are often hidden in processed foods.
- Do not eat the identified foods for at least two weeks.
- While eliminating the foods, watch how you feel, paying attention to any change in how you feel both physically and emotionally. It is helpful to keep a diary.
- If after your food elimination you're unsure of the results, try challenging yourself by eating a lot of the suspected food. Introduce suspected foods one at a time allowing 48 hours between foods. Note **any** reaction.

* Dairy includes milk, cheese, ice cream, yogurt, and anything made from milk. Some people only react to one form of dairy, such as milk, but not to others. During elimination, remove all forms of dairy. On the reintroduction challenge, test them one at a time.

** It is possible to react to any food, but these are the most common.

Treatment

Permanently eliminating foods you are severely allergic to is sometimes necessary for your health. Improving immune, digestive and detoxification function with a detoxification and rejuvenation program often reduces food sensitivities. Your *PW* doctor can help you with this process of healing.

Allergies and sensitivities are serious health problems. Discovering hidden allergens can dramatically improve a person's physical and mental health.

18. Avoid unproven detox treatments

Colonic Warning
Why **I do not** recommend colonics.

My oath as a doctor is to first "Do no harm." I take that oath seriously. I also believe in using therapies that have scientific validity.

What is a colonic? (Sometimes called colonic irrigation or colon hydrotherapy.)

The patient lies on a table. A tube is inserted in their rectum. Water (sometimes with additional minerals, good bacteria, or other components.) flows into the colon from a warming tank. The patient is instructed to hold the solution as long as comfortable. A clear outlet tube allows the patient and practitioner (usually not a doctor) to observe what is being removed from the colon. The inflow and release of solution continues for 30-60 minutes until the solution is clear.

No good science
In researching colonics I could find no supporting scientific studies. Their usefulness is only supported by testimonials ("I felt great"). Testimonials are sometimes valuable, but I'm always cautious when a therapy only has testimonial support. Doctors, celebrities, and others are often paid to endorse products.

When you read the history and listen to proponents of colonics it comes down to two main points:

1. If a person is constipated, they feel better when their bowels are emptied.

I agree. Constipation is a very real problem that compromises a person's health and needs to be treated. However, I disagree that colonics are a safe and effective way of treating constipation. There are safe and effective alternatives.

2. Sick people have colons that are lined with layers of sludge that need to be washed away with colonics.

I strongly disagree. If a person's colon was lined with layers of waste matter they would not be able to absorb nutrients or balance electrolytes and they would quickly die. Furthermore, if you ask a gastroenterologist who performs hundreds of colonoscopies (essentially looking inside the colon with a tiny camera) about "layers of sludge" they will say they never see such a thing. Layers of sludge is a **myth** that is perpetuated by proponents of colonics. I challenge them to show photographic proof, not imaginative drawings.

What is normal bowel function?
Many doctors ignore the normal functioning of the bowels. I've had patients who tell me their MD says it's normal to only have 1 or 2 bowel movements a week.

I disagree, based on the physiology of the bowels and population studies.

Physiology
When we eat food it stretches our stomach. That sends a signal to the brain that then sends a signal to the intestines to start peristalsis – the wave-like motion that moves food through our digestive system. This results in a bowel movement 30-90 minutes after eating.

Population studies
People who eat traditional diets (high fiber, no processed foods) tend to have three bowel movements per day; one after each meal. These people also have fewer health problems,

including hemorrhoids, gallstones, acne and varicose veins. Varicose veins and hemorrhoids are made worse by straining to move the bowels.

Okay, if you agree that three bowel movements per day triggered by a natural physiologic process are normal, how do colonics fit? Not at all.

Colonic Safety Concerns

There have been very few reported cases of problems caused by colonics. However, I do have two major concerns:

- Potential introduction of **harmful bacteria** because of poor maintenance and knowledge of hygiene. There have been reported cases of this causing illness.

- **Distention of the colon** caused by the stretching of the colon muscles. Colonic advocates say that colonics do the opposite; that they tone the muscles. However, they have no proof of this. They have never done a study to prove their point. On the other hand, logic says that if you insert large quantities of a liquid into a soft tube it will stretch. I say, why take a chance when there are safer, natural alternatives.

Colonics & laxatives: Short-term solutions for long-term problems

Colonics are a semi-surgical method of stimulating the bowel to move. Laxatives are a chemical method for stimulating bowel evacuation. Certainly a person who is constipated will feel better after a colonic or laxative, but that does not mean it's in their long-term health interest.

The healthy approach to constipation is to provide the nutrients that allow for a natural elimination of waste matter;

drink plenty of water, eat a fiber-rich diet, and supply vitamins and minerals.

If you are constipated or have other digestive problems, avoid quick and potentially dangerous therapies. Talk to your **Pure Wellness** (**PW**) physician about safe, natural ways of improving your health.

Foot pads and baths – unproven

Pads that attach to the bottom of your feet and "detox" foot baths have not been shown to remove toxins from the body. It would not be difficult to prove the effectiveness of these therapies if they worked. Patients could simply be tested before and after treatment for levels of toxins in their bodies. I have seen no supportive scientific evidence of their effectiveness.

Why use unproven therapies when scientifically supported therapies exist?

19. *Pure Weight Loss* when you don't have a PWC near you – email & phone consults

Ideally you have a doctor near you that understands healthy nutrition and detoxification who can help you with your health and weight issues. If not, **PWC** provides phone and email consultations. For the latest on how to participate, as well as pricing, go to ***www.PureWellnessCenters.com***.

Section VI

Conclusion
&
BioMarker Record

"The less you allow corporations to control your food intake and the more personal direction you follow, the healthier you will become. Your goal is not to be perfect in how you eat, but to be perfectly happy with what you eat."

Tom Ballard, ND

20. Conclusion

Your body is an ecological system, just as is the earth. If your goal is healthy weight control - weight loss for life – then you recognize that your weight and health are connected.

The two most important issues affecting most people's health are **environmental toxins and nutritional deficiencies** (genetics play a minor role for most people). We know this because research finds that everyone carries a load of toxic chemicals and is deficient in several food factors.

We also know there is a direct correlation between toxins, deficiencies, and **chronic health problems** such as diabetes, heart disease, fatigue, and **obesity**.

Evaluating the last fifty years of weight-loss tricks - low calorie and low fat diets, fat blockers, calorie counting, appetite suppressants, and stimulants – demonstrate a 95 percent failure rate over five years. In other words, only five percent successfully lose weight and keep it off. Clearly these gimmicks , as popular as they are, don't work. In fact, they usually **trigger yo-yo dieting and weight gain.**

Successful fat loss is the result of:

- **Removing** environmental toxins that slow your ability to burn calories.
- **Rejuvenating** your body with the nutrients it requires to produce energy and control appetite.

Note I said FAT loss. Other programs promote muscle and water loss, but what you want to lose is fat.

The ***Pure Weight Loss*** program is designed to support your weight loss through detoxification and rejuvenation. It is grounded in the latest science and is easy to incorporate into your life. True, your life will change. As you feel energized and see your body transforming, you'll be inspired to take further control of your diet and life.

Yes, this will take time. Just as you didn't reach your current weight overnight, it will take weeks, sometimes months, to achieve your goals. This is what it means to rejuvenate your body – the fundamental improvement in cell and organ function that transforms your health and stops the downward spiral into chronic disease and obesity.

With ***Pure Weight Loss*** you will be:

- **Eating** delicious, healthy meals, loaded with detoxifying and rejuvenating nutrients.
- Drinking a ***Pure Weight-Loss* shake** that stimulates cellular rejuvenation and controls food cravings.
- Enjoying **activities** that stimulate fat breakdown.
- **Supplementing** missing vitamins and minerals.
- Relaxing with our exclusive **Mind/Body Detoxification**.
- Monitoring your **BioMarkers** (weight, percent fat, water, and muscle) and **Free Radicals**.
- Achieving your weight and health goals with the **support** of your **PW** doctor.

Thank you for considering **Pure *Weight Loss***.
Our goal is your health!
Tom Ballard, RN, ND.

21. BioMarker Record

Name: _____ Goals: 6 wk _____ one yr_____

Date						
Weight						
Fat %						
Water%						
MuscleMass						
Muscle %						
BMR						
Met. Age						
BMI						
Waist/Hip						
Energy						
Free Rads						

Date						
Weight						
Fat %						
Water%						
MuscleMass						
Muscle %						
BMR						
Met. Age						
BMI						
Waist/Hip						
Energy						
Free Rads						

Body composition is a result of lifestyle choices and is under your control. If you have questions, please consult with your **PWL** doctor or see us at **www.PureWellnessCenters.com**.

Proof

4586462

Made in the USA
Charleston, SC
15 February 2010